THE OIL-DISPERSION BATH

Its Natural Basis and Practical Use

Werner Junge

Translated by Gladys Hahn
and edited by Gerald Karnow

All Rights Reserved

Copyright 1980, 2025

ISBN: 978-1-957569-47-5

Published by
MERCURY PRESS
an imprint of SteinerBooks
PO Box 58
Hudson, New York 12534
www.steinerbooks.org

THE OIL-DISPERSION BATH

Its Natural Basis and
Practical Use

Table of Contents

INTRODUCTION

It was 35 years ago that the attempt was made to bring to reality the idea of a therapeutic oil bath. We would now like to review the result of this work and to consider possible uses of this still very new method of hydrotherapy.

The history of this specific therapy goes back to indications which Rudolf Steiner gave in 1920. In "Spiritual Science and Medicine", Lecture 15, he pointed to the inner relationship of the oil-forming process in nature to the warmth nature of man; that warmth is the carrier and the agent of the spiritual processes in nature and in man. If there is weakness in the warmth organism, that causes a slackening of spiritual activity, of ego activity.

All therapy depends upon the diagnosis of the cause of the illness. With the nineteenth century came an end of old traditions that formerly had influenced medical thought: traditions of an all-embracing Nature. A knowledge was lost of forces which had earlier been experienced: forces that work from outside the earth into earthly and human relations. Since then, the medical thought oriented to natural science limits itself to a physical-material basis for life processes. The human organism is finally regarded as only a mechanism - albeit a very complicated one. Thus not only has the living relationship, indeed the most elementary interdependence of man and nature, become seriously endangered: the inability to return to a meaningful approach to the healing forces of nature, i.e. in the true sense of good health, has become increasingly clear.

Therefore Rudolf Steiner's research into the nature of man was fundamental for a true understanding of pathology and therapy. In 1917 in his book "Von Seelenratseln ("Riddles of the Soul") he spoke for the first time of "the threefold human organism". This was the key to a new understanding of the living principles active in nature and man.

It was Goethe who discovered the law of polarity and growth that underlies all life. Rudolf Steiner pointed in a concrete way to cosmic and terrestrial forces which are active as a "polarity" within evolving nature and man.

In his investigations of the organic basis for "the soul in man", he was able to point to the three systems of the organism:

> The Nerve Sense System - bearer of consciousness and
> thinking;

> The Metabolic-Limb System - carrier of the life of instinct
> and will;

-binding these together and harmonizing them -
The Rhythmic System (Blood Circulation and Breathing) -
carrier of the life of feeling.

Man's trichotomy - spirit, soul, body - is thereby given its physiological-psychological coordination.

Thus the spiritual nature of the human ego was recognized; the body as expression of the physical; the soul (feeling- and life-organism) as mediator between spiritual and physical, between cosmos and earth.

Of course, the higher members of man's being lie beyond the scope of a purely external scrutiny; even so, we must give them their proper place and due consideration if only for the sake of a useful working hypothesis. Physical organism and ego organism confront each other as a polarity just as do matter and spirit. If the function of the life-and feeling-organism is to mediate between the two opposite members, the physical and the spiritual, then the archetypal Threefold nature of man (body, soul and spirit) can be brought back again - with new significance - into human knowledge and into therapeutic thought.

I.   THE INNER IDENTITY OF THE WARMTH PROCESS AND EGO-ACTIVITY

In the lecture mentioned above, in the course "Spiritual Science and Medicine", Rudolf Steiner describes man's spiritual nature, his ego-being, as a cosmic entity that works as a peripheral force - as "the most completely extraterrestrial" force - into and upon his central physical forces. This "cosmic ego-being" finds its correspondence in the warmth processes of nature. In the plant it is the oil- forming processes that bring the cosmic being of the plant from the environment into visible appearance. In man this same task, which relates to the incarnation of a human being, is performed by his warmth organism. If therefore the ego-organization, that is, man's warmth organism is weakened - which is the case, for instance, in diabetes mellitus - that is a sign of the weakening of the spiritual warmth process (the environment forces). Therefore - in Rudolf Steiner's own words - we can "relate the ego to the oil-forming process. The best way to do this is by finding a way to intro-duce finely dispersed oil into a bath; then the patient can be given oil-bath treatments. This is something that would be highly desirable..."   (from Lecture 15)

II.   KNOWLEDGE OF MAN AS THE FOUNDATION FOR OIL-BATH THERAPY

We have already pointed out the most important fact to be considered in making arrangements for oil baths: that is, the relation of the oil-producing process in nature to the ego-activity in man. There can be no thought of using oil as a ponderable substance, as it is used, for instance, in massage-rubbing. Rudolf Steiner's indication was to attempt to develop an oil process in water by finely dispersing the oil. Again it is not a question of simply dissolving the oil in water, as one can do without further ado by using emulsifiers. By this method the oil-process is nullified. In customary emulsification one can no longer speak of oil.

Quite another way to spread oil through water to the finest possible degree, is offered by the idea of the whirlpool. When a whirlpool occurs in water, an extraordinarily high speed of rotation develops immediately at the center. And related to that, a partial vacuum (low pressure) appears. The physicist Eck has established by his research that this event is not just a matter of a difference in pressure, but of "negative pressure", that is, suction.

The whirlpool we need is brought about with the help of a device [i.e., a jet pump - Tr.] that is placed as a whirling body in the path of rapidly flowing water. Above the whirlpool center is a capillary nozzle leading from an oil containing reservoir. The water running through the device sucks the oil down into the whirlpool. The oil comes into the region of negative pressure and undergoes a so-called evaporation. It is led over from its fluid state into a vapor condition - entirely by the speed of the swirling water. This transformation into vapor is otherwise only brought about by warmth.

Through the change of state the oil now has the tendency to revert to its original condition, that is, to condense again. But by passing through the whirlpool the oil has become homogeneously distributed in the water; it cannot now condense without some further process. The water has become thoroughly permeated by an oil-mist. This mist can be rendered visible with light rays. (Tyndall effect.) Despite the finest dispersion the contrast between oil and water still exists. But due to the forces of repulsion that are active on all sides, the buoyancy of the oil is neutralized and the oil remains bound to the water as a mist in suspension. Yet the oil has the natural tendency to free itself again from the water, to condense. And the first opportunity to do so is presented by the body of the bath patient. Just as, for example, a salt solution can only crystallize if an external impetus sets it in motion, similarly condensation of the oil is initiated by the body of the bath patient.

Perhaps this gives a picture of how we have tried to solve the problem of using the oil-forming process in an "oil-dispersion bath".

And now, having given this bath to patients, can we report objective results which allow us to conclude that the bath does have a positive effect on the haan warmth organism?

In the case of diabetes mellitus, Dr. Steiner gave the following explanation of its cause: the individual's ego-organization is not working in his organism with complete force. The ego is the spiritual member of the human organism; it has to have a carrier or agent to be able to work right down into the physical body. And the warmth organism must be recognized as this carrier for the spiritual activity of the ego in the organism.

In a human being there is always an intensive life process to correspond to an intensive warmth process. Accordingly, in a patient whose ego-organization is not active throughout his entire body, it would be logical to find low temperatures in body areas that are so impoverished. In fact this symptom of low temperatures appears so frequently that it is so often spoken of as "atrophy" of the warmth organism.

III.   THE EFFECTS OF OIL-DISPERSION BATHS ON THE HUMAN WARMTH ORGANISM

The first and also the most general effect of these baths that we observe in a patient is a warmth reaction. This develops very subtly, but it can be followed with a thermometer. Taking the patient's temperature under the tongue, one can observe this warmth process unfolding during the bath. One realizes from this warmth reaction that the ego-activity begins to be stimulated. This is an active process, and not just a damming-up of warmth caused by the external temperature of the bath water. That it really has to do with an active process is especially evident when the body temperature during the bath even rises above the temperature of the bath water. The oil-dispersion baths have this characteristic, that due to the increasing warmth of his blood, the patient does not feel the actual coolness of the bath water. Nor does he feel the gradual cooling-off of the water, which can be as much as 2° C.   (35.6° F.).

It is also possible to observe the rhythmic relation of circulation and breathing, especially in cases where it has been disturbed by illness. The oil-dispersion baths -are not contra-indicated even in cases of severe circulatory disturbances. On the contrary, in a short time the ratio of pulse to respiration begins to normalize, and this persists after the bath.

In cases of severe circulatory disturbances, especially in the lower legs, already after the second or third bath a clearing of the lividity along the veins has been observed and even a decrease of the hyper-pigmentation. Repeatedly in cases of lower legs ready for amputation, the circulatory disturbance was overcome and the amputation avoided.

In one case of a hand injured by a circular saw, it was observed that the severe venous bleeding stopped after three minutes in an oil-dispersion bath. After a subsequent sequence of baths, the wound healed well with extensive regeneration of the skin, so that scar tissue was minimal.

Especially informative are the reports of leg amputees. One war victim with an above knee amputation was still having phantom pains after twenty years. But he felt only the joints of the leg that had been removed. In the course of his bath treatments consciousness of the entire leg returned. The feeling of pain was replaced by a feeling of warmth.

Another patient, 63 years old, came to us after an above knee amputation. She was very conscious of the leg that was no longer there, but it seemed like a foreign body. When she was lying in bed she felt that the leg hung down vertically beneath her and that it was cold. She was unable to alter this feeling of the leg's position. After six oil-dispersion baths she could move the phantom leg at will, and now she had the feeling that the leg was warm. Her general health improved correspondingly.

Besides the cardiovascular illnesses the various rheumatic disturbances are an area in which the oil-dispersion baths can be used with great benefit.

The question arises: how can this wide range of application by means of one single therapeutic measure be explained? For an answer we must first investigate the substance, oil, and inquire how it is formed in plants, for instance.

IV.   THE OIL-FORMING PROCESS AND THE THREEFOLD NATURE OF PLANTS

There are certain plants that develop their oil formation particularly strongly, and therefore are called "oil plants". Disregarding them for a moment, we can assert that there is an oil-forming process in every blossoming plant; and that it is a process necessary to the plant s life.

In the formation of every seed, oil appears in the germ. What task does this oil have in the life of the plant?

First there are watery saps in the plant. For these to be changed to oil, it is necessary above all for warmth to be active. Oil shows itself to be a substance in which warmth and light are stored to a high degree as imponderable elements.

The plant has no inner organ for keeping its life processes in rhythm, as do animal and man. Nevertheless it does possess certain rhythmic processes that can be compared to breathing and circulation. However, the rhythmic cycles are not controlled by the plant itself. They are created by influences outside the plant. The plant's life is entirely dependent upon the daily and seasonal cycles of the year. The plant is suspended in the inter-action between earth and cosmos.

For the plant, earth and cosmos create a polarity of active forces that determine its life. But the terrestrial and extraterrestrial forces also need the mediation of a third category of forces for their interaction and their organic formation activity.

The extraterrestrial forces that work into the plant from outer space bring about an acceleration of its life processes. This can be observed particularly in the movement of sap. When sap rises in the trees, this is not due to pressure at the roots, but to a suction process that is accomplished within the tree by cosmic forces. This process also explains the fact that the speed of movement of rising sap increases as the tree grows in height, and does not end even in the tops of the highest giant trees. Most of the water taken in through the roots is evaporated; that means, the sap actually rises beyond the top of the tree into the atmosphere.

One realizes from observing this phenomenon that the cosmic forces, the forces from outside the earth, would dissolve the substance of the plants and would suck them away from the earth if the earth forces were not exerting a contrary influence.

Quite different in character are the earth forces. They predominate in the seed formation. They work from the earth outwards. They want to centralize the plant as in a point. With this is connected a condensing of substance and a slackening of movement within the plant. If the life process were finally to reach a complete standstill in the seed, it would have become a dead mineral out of which no new plant could develop.

Now what is there in the plant that on the one hand restrains the dissolving of its substance and on the other hand restrains the densifying of its substance which would otherwise bring the plant's life process to an end?

What we are looking for cannot lie in the cosmic or earth forces, for the influences coming from these opposite directions would tear the plant to pieces.

Although a plant does not possess inner organs, there are nevertheless organic processes going on within it. And it is in these "plant-organ-processes" that one recognizes activities that synthesize the polarity earth-cosmos. The plant can withstand the suction-and-dissolving of the peripheral forces by its formation of resin. It can withstand the complete cessation of its life process which the earth forces would bring about, by its formation of oil in the seed. The distinctive quality of oil is its inner mobility, and that is the basis of its vitality.

It is through the germ oil in the seed that the plant's life is maintained through the successive stages of its growth.

Resin, ethereal oil and fatty oil: these three substances are the product of a special category of forces which together with the cosmic and earth forces form a triad:

Cosmic Warmth - forces from the periphery (dissolution of substance)

Ethereal Oil Fatty Oil   rhythmic balancing
                Resin - earth forces
                (condensing of substance)

This three fold character of the warmth process in plants corresponds to the threefold character of the human organism:

Nerve-Sense System
Rhythmic System (blood-respiration) Metabolic-Limb System

And these have as their foundation the three members of the human being:

Spirit - Soul (life) - Body

In the plant as in man, it is the warmth processes that bring the spiritual entity - plant being or human ego - down into physical corporeality. And the substances that carry the warmth are the oils.

We have tried to show that resin and oil are the physical manifestation of a special category of forces that bring the polar forces of cosmos and earth to a synthesis in the plant. Only then is its development possible. The resin- and oil-forming process creates a middle sphere between earthly and cosmic forces. The really central position is held by the oil-forming process.

In the resins the cosmic warmth process comes to an end. In the oil-forming process the polarity of forces between earth and cosmos appears mirrored once more in the phenomena/formation of fatty oils and etheral oils. Fatty and ethereal oils are fundamentally different. Ethereal oils are related in their activity to the cosmic forces; fatty oils unfold their activity in the life realm.

In the use of oil for therapy it is possible to cope with the enormous diversity of human illnesses by appropriate mixtures of fatty and ethereal oils

V.   THE PHENOMENA OF WATER

To understand fully how the oil-dispersion bath works, we must first make a few observations about water.

The usual impression that water makes on an observer is that of movement. As one observes the movement one notices that water has the capacity to transform all influences to which it is exposed into rhythmic processes. This is seen most clearly in the way waves are formed.

Wave crest-and-trough present a rhythmic pendulum movement around a middle position which represents the ideal surface. (See H. Bauer, Physical Phenomena of Water. Wala Medical Laboratory, Eckwalden 1960) When the moving surface comes to rest, then it reflects. This capacity to reflect is, as it were, an external sign of the inner readiness of water to take in all instreaming forces and give them out again.

Careful observation reveals the further fact that water not only forms an outer surface, but further more every movement in its flow also creates inner surfaces. Water is therefore not an undifferentiated body; rather, it is structured within itself in the form of surfaces. (See Th. Schwenk: The Sensible Chaos. Verlag Freies Geistesleben)

The most interesting phenomenon to be found when investigating how a particular surface comes about in water, is the whirlpool formation. In a circling movement of flowing water one observes that the speed of flow is increased, the closer the flow comes to the center of its movement. This causes the surface to sink in, and a typical funnel form is created. The important aspect of this is that the whirling of the water develops a suction force. All the water that arrives in the funnel is pulled down to the bottom with great speed.

It is essential to see that the cause of this suction force in the whirlpool does not lie in any mechanical conditions, such as, for instance, friction between the fast-flowing water and the air. The real cause is something very different. At first the water has been filling a three-dimensional space;' then in the area of the whirlpool there comes a partial breakdown of the spatial three-dimensional condition. And the result is a qualitative transformation from static to dynamic forces: in place of pressure there are now suction forces. The forming of surfaces, especially in the whirlpool, reveals the true nature of water.

A vessel filled with water creates the impression that water also has three dimensions. But the water is only held together by the vessel - and that is just as true for a riverbed, lakebed or oceanbed. The water appears to have a spatial three-dimensional form. However, without a vessel it spreads immediately into a two-dimensional surface, because water actually does not have a third dimension, Therefore we should pay special attention again to the surface-forming phenomenon when a whirlpool develops.

We have pointed cut that the form created by the whirlpool is typical. Regardless of the size of a whirlpool, the geometry of the funnel wall is always the same. It is shaped by an infinity of tangent cones, whose surface area is constant. When a whirlpool is formed, beginning with a random circular motion, then the enclosed surface can already be thought of as a cone, with zero height (or depth) and a definite radius. As the whirlpool formation continues to develop, the height increases. Correspondingly, the radius must become smaller, hence the surface area remains constant. If the height should reach infinity, the radius could be zero. That would mean, the whirlpool has been transformed from a two-dimensional surface to a one-dimensional form: its surface has taken the form of a ray.

The transformation of spatial, three-dimensional character through a two-dimensional form to one dimension brings about the development of dynamics, of a world of moving forces. Expressed more exactly, the introduction of dynamics into the world of space nullifies it.

Of course, in nature the ultimate form never is manifest as it can be constructed in thought. Associated with the whirlpool is a wave formation around the whirlpool form; the wave moves on a spiral path This wave formation brings a force into action that prevents the whirlpool from actually becoming a ray. The spiraling wave cuts the whirl-pool off at a definite place.

Let us go back to the threefold human being, the entelechy of body, soul and spirit. As we observed the life processes of the plant we had to differentiate between earthly-and-cosmic forces which form a polarity, and the forces which mediate between these polar extremes, forces without which there could be no plant life at all. And so we found in nature also a threefoldness of active forces which corresponds to the human picture.

Our study of water has led us to find within the spatial three-dimensional earth-body a world of moving forces through whose activity the world of space can experience a reduction to one dimension. Are there also phenomena that suggest the possibility of reaching non-dimensionality?

VI.   WARMTH, THE MEDIATOR BETWEEN PONDERABLE AND IMPONDERABLE FORCES

At the beginning of this study we said we would try to give the background of a certain therapeutic procedure. Now we must show that it is in the realm of non-dimensionality that a*. finds the source of healing forces.

In the transition from three to two dimensions forces of movement appeared. The intensity of these forces was further increased in the transition from two dimensions to one dimension. Therefore it follows that upon reaching non-dimensionality the most intense energy of movement must appear. The natural phenomenon that leads the way into this realm is warmth. Warmth can be described as a boundary phenomenon between the ponderable realm of matter and the imponderable realm of spirit; physically expressed, between pressure phenomena and suction phenomena. H. Bauer has pointed to the phenomena of drop formation and capillary action as evidence of this same tendency to polarity in water. Warmth is the active element in the boundary realm between pressure and suction. (See Rudolf Steiner, Natural Scientific Course 1920, Lecture 10.)

Warmth holds the same position in the physical realm as the oil-forming process holds in the organic realm of the plant world. And just as there are opposite tendencies at work in the forming of fatty and ethereal oils, so there are opposite tendencies at work in warmth. According to whether it moves in the direction of pressure activity or suction activity, it will bring about processes of materialization or dematerialization. Materialization and dematerialization correspond to a rarification and an intensification of the forces of movement, which manifest as processes of deceleration and acceleration. When the process of deceleration comes to an end, that is. when it comes finally to a standstill, then the maximum spatial-material condition is reached. An infinite acceleration would bring about the opposite condition.

In the threefold human being the ego is the spiritual member. To continue the foregoing line of thought, spirit and ego now appear as the "most completely cosmic" entity, the "most completely un-spatial", as the realm of non-dimensionality, out of which all formative impulses of the living-soul-world as well as of the spatial-mineralworld flow on the waves of rhythm.

Healing forces work out of the spirit into the world by way of warmth, oil and water. The oil-dis^Persion bath offers the possibility to continue this path through water, oil, blood, warmth to the ego of man. Because of the intimate connection of the human organism with the cosmic forces, the ego is enabled to give a powerful impulse again to the life processes and to establish long-lost health once more.

VII.   APPLICATION AND TECHNIQUE OF THE OIL-DISPERSION BATH

In using the oil-dispersion baths it is very important to control the bath temperatures precisely. They must be measured constantly. They may not be simply approximated.

Disorders of the cardiovascular and the nervous system require cool baths. (32°-34°C.=F.89.6°-93.2°) Metabolic disorders require a higher temperature. However, every patient should feel comfortable in his bath, so that he neither sweats nor feels chilled. That means, every single patient requires his individual bath temperature. To begin with, until this individual temperature is known, it is better to make the bath too cool rather than too
warm, because it is easier and more pleasant for the patient to change from a cooler to a warmer temperature. Baths that are too warm can disturb the desired delicate reaction of warmth. The length of the bath depends upon this warmth reaction, which usually occurs after five to fifteen minutes. An oil-dispersion bath should not be continued longer than twenty minutes.

Following the bath the patient is wrapped warmly without being dried and rests for at least one hour. He is wrapped in bath towels and blankets which fit snuggly around him. Then the warmth process, already stimulated in the bath, can continue without interruption, so that after a few minutes the patient again has a pleasant sensation of being permeated by warmth.

It will sometimes happen that at the beginning of bath treatments a patient experiences no warmth reaction during the bath. Today this lack of reaction is a familiar situation. In most cases, however, a rapid warmth reaction occurs afterwards during the resting time. If the inner warmth does not come, either during the bath or during the rest, even after several baths have been given, that is an indication that among other things another oil should be used, one that corresponds better to the patient's needs.

It can also happen, even when the most appropriate oil is used, that at first there is an exacerbation in the illness. Even if this happens, the effect of the bath is to be judged as being positive if the ratio of pulse to respiration was normal or possibly even improved during the bath. Another positive sign is if a fresh color suffuses the skin of the face during the bath. This is particularly impressive with cancer patients, when the grey, lifeless appearing skin changes color. In the color of the lips one can also immediately recognize a stimulated blood-circulation.

Far more common than an initial worsening of a disorder, is the experience of temporary improvement in the patient.

The following observation is often made: especially if the first bath has produced a strong effect, the effect of the subsequent baths can occasionally be considerably weaker. How are these things reconciled?

Today, even in conventional medicine "health" is defined as the condition of homeostasis.

This is considered to be the balance of rhythmic interactions between opposing forces in the organism. Health depends upon the processes working toward this balance. It represents a neutral condition of which the human being is not conscious.

For a person who is ill the greatest changes will occur with the first oil dispersion bath. As the condition normalizes the subjective impressions also change.

We have mentioned that the different oils possess different qualities. They present a great variety of forces and one must be able to differentiate between them. The difference in their effects is the result of the different places in the plant where they were formed. For instance, a blossom oil works in a different way on the human organism than a root oil. The blossom oil affects the ego by way of the metabolic system, while the root oil effects the ego by way of the nerve-sense system.

It can happen that a satisfactory balance is achieved only by using several oils at different times. But as long as the therapist is still working his way into the use of this bath method he will attain a broad view and certainty in the procedures more quickly if he uses single oils at first and studies their effects.

Technical Procedures of the Oil-Dispersion Bath:

The finest dispersion of oil in water is accomplished without having to use any emulsifier whatsoever. A persistent binding of oil and water is brought about by virtue of a device that creates a whirlpool in the water. In the center of the whirlpool a vacuum forms. The capillary nozzle of an oil reservoir projects into this low pressure zone. The water pouring through this device is sucked into the whirlpool. Because of the low pressure a so-called cold evaporation takes place. Thus the oil is subject to a new physical condition. This transformation of the oil, together with the high speed of movement of the water, brings about an exceedingly fine homogeneous dispersion of the oil in the entire tub of water.

All other attempts at dispersing oil in water, for instance by pressure from a penetrating jet of water, have failed and furthermore produced negative therapeutic results.

For use of the oil-dispersion apparatus 3-5ccm of oil are needed for a full bath.

VIII.   RHYTHMIC UNDER-WATER BRUSH MASSAGE

The under-water brush massage has been developed as a supplementary treatment to the oil-dispersion bath, to stimulate peripheral blood-circulation. It is used in cases of paresis, strokes (CVAs), arthroses, hypo- and hypertension and disturbances in the peripheral circulation.

Two brushes are used: broad, flat brushes of "Biberach" form, with the piassava bristles, that is, palm leaf fibers, finely cut for this particular purpose. All other bristles soon become too soft in the oil-dispersion bath.

Circular strokes are used around the joints, and on other parts long straight strokes. The latter are always made toward the heart and along the entire length of the limb. One does not then carry the stroke back to its starting point, but stops and repeats the same stroke in the same direction. Each stroke is repeated from three to five times, until a hyperemic response is observed. A brush is held in each hand and the movement is carried out with both hands, either simultaneously or alternating. order: The parts of the body are brushed in the following

At first the patient lies in the tub on his back. Always begin with the -

Right Foot - On the top of the foot, straight strokes upward to the ankle. Cross to the outer edge (very strongly); the small front arch; the heel (very strongly) in circular movement. Then the ankle with both brushes at the same time, inner and outer with circular brushing.

Right Lower Leg - Straight strokes up to the knee, on the shin side and calf side.

Right Knee - Circular strokes clockwise.

Right Upper Leg - Straight strokes up to hip, all around. Right Hip - Circular strokes outward.

Left Leg - Brush in same way as right, but make the circular strokes opposite to those on the right leg.

Right Arm - Long straight strokes from the back of the hand to shoulder joint, and from palm to armpit.

Right Shoulder Joint - Circular movement, including the right shoulder blade.

Left Arm - Same as right arm; circular strokes around left shoulder in opposite direction to right shoulder.

Abdomen - First, straight strokes from the symphysis pubis to the right upper quadrant,

13

horizontal to the left upper quadrant, then downwards to the symphysis, increasing the pressure of the brush with this last downward stroke. Then with both brushes circular movement clockwise around navel.

Chest - Both brushes, one after the other over the breastbone, up to the collarbone, to right and left out to shoulder joints.

Next the patient sitting up in tub -

Lower Back - Fist, horizontal lemniscate strokes, then straight strokes the length of the spine up to shoulders; circular strokes around the seventh cervical vertebra.

For patients who have difficulty moving, the brush massage should end here. Other patients now lie in tub on the stomach.

Along the segmental tracts, right and left simultaneously, from outer side of feet in a straight stroke to between the shoulder blades - three to five times.

Then from inner side of feet to lower back, likewise in straight strokes.

Finally, both shoulder blades, circling inwards.

LIST OF THE DISPERSION OILS, WITH INDICATIONS FOR THEIR USE

Aconitum e tub. 5%, oil
> Nerve pains of every kind, for instance, head and facial neuralgia, lumbago.

Aesculus e sem. 5%, oil
> Varicose symptom - complex, rheumatic illnesses, rheumatic conditions, as adjunct in intervertebral syndromes.

Anise, ether. oil 5%
> Catarrhal symptoms of the respiratory passages and of alimentary canal.

Archangelica, ether. oil 1%
> Illnesses of the lymphatic system, especially in lung area and area of alimentary canal.

Arnica e flor. 5%, oil
> Rheumatic ailments and traumatic muscle and joint disturbances.

Berberis e rad. 10%, oil
> Sinus affections, functional disturbances of liver and gall bladder, also of kidney-bladder tract.

Betula e fol. 5%, oil
> Rheumatic ailments; to stimulate excretion via the kidneys

Calamus, ether. oil 5%
> Weak digestion, meteorism, edema.

Calendula e flor. 10%, oil
> Inflammatory processes of the skin.

Camphor 5%, oil
> Circulatory weaknesses with feelings of cold; rheumatic constitution.

Carum Carvi, ether. oil 5'
> Digestive weaknesses, meteorism.

Chamomilla e flor. 10%, oil
> Inflammatory and spastic conditions in stomach and intestinal area and urinary tract; especially valuable in pediatrics.

Citrus, ether. oil 107
> Tissue weakness and resulting symptoms such as prolapse, varicose veins; an adjunct in bronchial asthma.

Equisetum ex herba 5%, oil
> Disturbances in kidney-bladder area, especially with insufficient excretion.

Eucalyptus, ether. oil 10% Colds, hypersecretion.

Foeniculum ether oil 10%
> Digestive weakness, meteorism.

Hypericum ex herba 5%, oil
> General constitutional weakness, especially useful in pediatrics (enuresis nocturna); difficulties in going to sleep, injuries, sprains.

Juniperus comm., ether oil 5%
> Disturbances in calcium metabolism.

Lapps e rad. 5%, oil
> Dyspepsia; connective tissue disturbances.

Lavendula, ether. oil 10%
> Degenerative symptoms in nervous system; multiple sclerosis, paralysis, tendency to faint; overwork, sleeplessness.

Levisticum e rad. 5%, oil
> Neuritis, polyneuritis, hyperchromic anemia.

Pure Linseed, oil
> Sclerosis; as adjunct in therapy of carcinoma, especially in postoperative treatment.

Melissa ex herbs 5%, oil
> Weakness of generative organs, dysmenorrhea, spasms, liver-gall bladder disorders.

Nicotiana e fol. 10%, oil
> Spasms of all kinds, particularly arterial, asthmatic and anginal conditions.

Oxalis e pl. tota 10%, oil
> Metabolic weakness, especially with tendency to form stones in liver, gall bladder and kidney regions; conditions following shock.

Passiflora ex herba 5%, oil Sleeplessness, restlessness.

Petroselinum, ether. oil 5%
> Spasms in kidney and bladder areas; anuria; enuresis nocturna.

Pinus pumilio, ether. oil 10%
> Respiratory illnesses; chronic bronchitis, scrofula, neuritis, obesity, plethora, stone forming in kidney and bladder areas.

Prunus spin. e flor. 5%, oil
> Conditions of exhaustion; general constitutional weakness, flaccidity of skin and of subcutaneous tissue.

Rheuma Bath oil
> Oil extracts from Betula (folia), Arnica (flores), Lappa (radix), Urtica dioeca (herba), Formica, 01. Anisi 0.35%
> Rheumatic illnesses of muscles and joints; sprains bruises; muscle pains from over-exertion.

Rosa e flor. 10%, oil
> Circulatory weakness and conditions of exhaustion, especially in convalescence.

Rosemarinus, ether. oil 10%
> Metabolic weakness, especially diabetes; hyper-tension, inadequate warmth formation, obesity.

Salvia, ether. oil 10%
> Excessive perspiration in puberty and menopause; respiratory illnesses.

Terebinthina laricina 10%, oil
> Hardening and mineralizing tendencies connected with ageing; ailments of the retina; stone-forming tendencies of kidney.

Thuja e summit. 5%, oil
> Tendency of excessive growth and inflammation of skin and mucous membranes; constitutional weakness.

Thyme, ether. oil 5%
>Colds and associated respiratory illnesses; bronchial spasms, rickets, Sudeck's syndrome.

Urtica dioeca ex herba 5%, oil
>Circulatory weakness, anemia, eczema, asthma, rheumatism, gout, general constitutional weakness.

Valeriana, ether. oil 1%
>Restlessness, sleeplessness, nervous exhaustion, cardiac unrest.

Viscum mall e planta tot 5%, oil
>Chronic polyarthritis, arthritis deformans; for treatment after radiation therapy - in some cases alternating with Solum uliginosum comp. bath sub-stance.

The oils mentioned in this list are prepared by Wala-Heilmittel, Dr. R. Hauschka OHG, 7325 Eckwaelden/Bad Boll and can be ordered through any pharmacy (in Germany). Linseed oil (Lini purum) is available in health food stores.

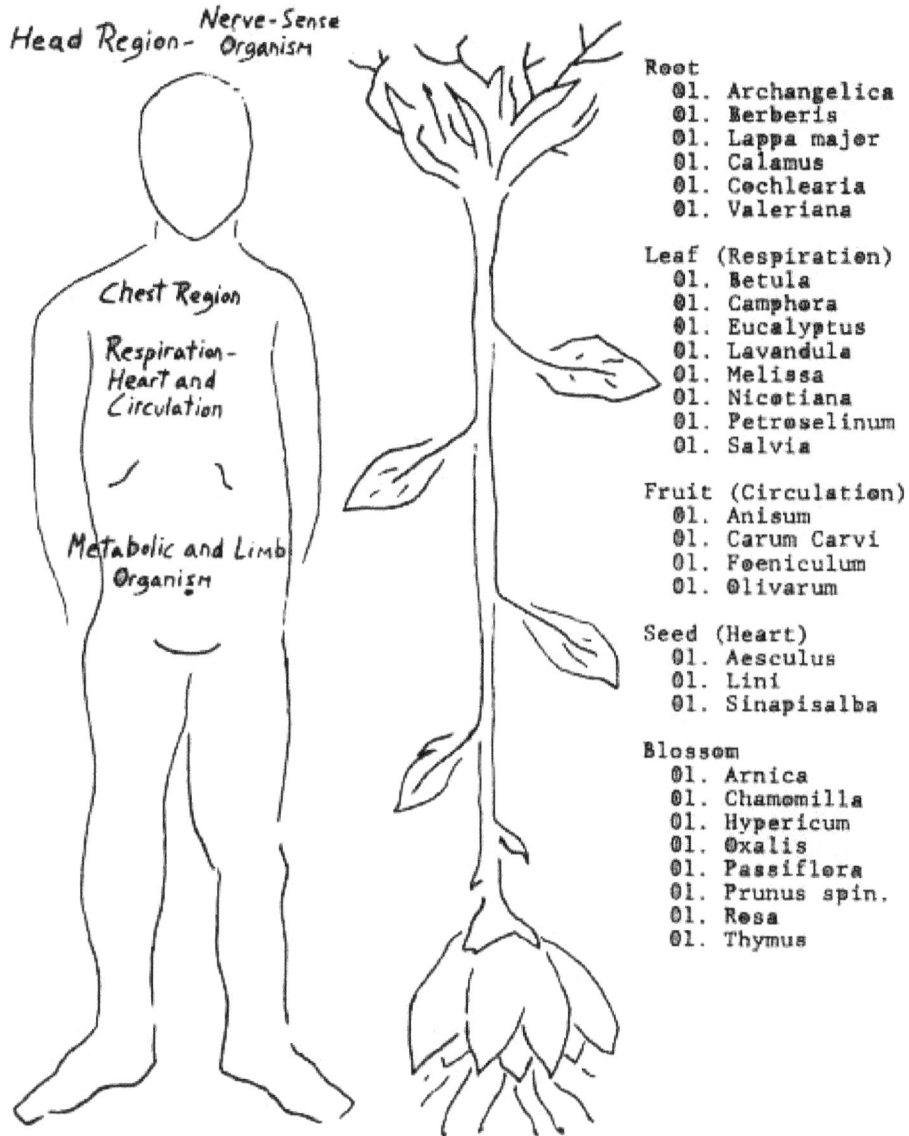

Areas of Oil Formation in the Plant
and its Relation to the Human Organism

Head Region— Nerve-Sense Organism

Chest Region

Respiration—
Heart and
Circulation

Metabolic and Limb
Organism

Root
  01. Archangelica
  01. Berberis
  01. Lappa major
  01. Calamus
  01. Cochlearia
  01. Valeriana

Leaf (Respiration)
  01. Betula
  01. Camphora
  01. Eucalyptus
  01. Lavandula
  01. Melissa
  01. Nicotiana
  01. Petroselinum
  01. Salvia

Fruit (Circulation)
  01. Anisum
  01. Carum Carvi
  01. Foeniculum
  01. Olivarum

Seed (Heart)
  01. Aesculus
  01. Lini
  01. Sinapisalba

Blossom
  01. Arnica
  01. Chamomilla
  01. Hypericum
  01. Oxalis
  01. Passiflora
  01. Prunus spin.
  01. Rosa
  01. Thymus

www.ingramcontent.com/pod-product-compliance
Lightning Source LLC
Chambersburg PA
CBHW080058280326

41934CB00014B/3361